Do Like Grandma Did:
A Guide to Clean Healthy Eating

by Alice W. Munyua,

Board Certified Family Nurse Practitioner

Alice W. Munyua

ISBN-10: 1-944662-04-9

ISBN-13: 978-1-944662-04-2

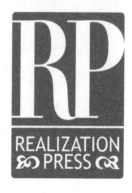

Cover Art by Annie Flood

Table of Contents

Disclaimer

This book is intended as a reference volume only, not as a medical manual. It is not a substitute for any treatment that may have been prescribed by your doctor. If you suspect that you have a medical problem, we urge you to seek medical help. Keep in mind that nutritional needs vary from person to person, depending upon age, sex, health status and total diet. The information discussed here is intended to help you make informed decisions about your diet and health.

Chapter 1
My Story

I grew up on a farm in Kenya close to the slopes of Aberdare Ranges. It is a hilly place where we grew coffee, tea and kept dairy cows. That was our livelihood. I came to the United States as a college student in my early 20s. My grandma who helped raise me stayed in Kenya. You might be wondering why my grandma's story is important to you. Hang on; I will explain.

As I have watched the world go crazy about gluten-free diets and the clean eating (healthy eating) movement, I realize that some people are just plain confused. People are spending money on things they should not be and putting themselves on dietary restrictions and none of it is helping. The obesity epidemic is not getting better and, as a matter of fact, it is getting worse. As I have watched all this confusion about eating, I just have to say something.

Clean eating is not a new concept. It's been around for decades. It's also easy and simple to do: You simply do like Grandma did and you will be eating clean every single day of your life. ***Eat Like Grandma Did***.

My grandma was a tall, beautiful, svelte woman. She was a force of energy and had a youthfulness about her. A well-known woman, she was sought after for advice on various things by her peers in the village. In terms of her health, there are some things that Grandma did and some things that she didn't do. She passed on that knowledge to my mother, who then passed it on to me. I have a feeling that your grandma might have done the same.

As a testimony to her life, my grandma passed away at the tender age of 94 years young, and she kept the same weight most of her adult life. She didn't take any medications and had no chronic medical issues like diabetes, hypertension or heart disease. She passed her wisdom about clean eating to my mother, who died as a result of in accident at the age of 74. Like my grandma, she didn't take any medications and had no chronic medical issues.

I am in my early 50s and at a perfect weight for my height. I do not take any medications other than Ibuprofen for tension headaches at times. I have no chronic medical issues and hope to be 94 years old someday and be like my grandma was.

Chapter 2
Where Did We Go Wrong?

Why is the obesity crisis what it is today? I am told that the problem started in the early 1970s when _someone_ told people that "fat makes people fat." What followed was a movement where people started avoiding fats like the plague. They began consuming large amounts of carbohydrates instead. Anything low-fat was considered good: low-fat peanut butter, low-fat muffins, low-fat bagels, low-fat cookies, low-fat cakes, etc. This information was not evidence-based, but people took it as the gospel truth. What everyone has failed to know was that in order for low-fat food to taste good, it has to have more sugar.

In 1978, the average American adult consumed 1,826 calories a day. Less than 42.6% was in carbohydrates (carbs), 40.5% was in fats and 16.5% was in proteins.

In 2006, the average American adult consumed 2,157 calories a day. Less than 49.9% was in carbs, 33.6% was in fats and 15.4% was in proteins.

In 2010, the average American adult consumed 2,400 calories a day. About 51% was in carbs, 33% was in fats and 16% was in proteins.

In 2014, the average American adult consumed 2,550 calories a day and about 52% of that was carbs, 33% was fats and 15% was protein.

I came to this country in the mid-1980s when the low-fat movement was in full swing. People consumed more and more calories as time went on. Today people consume nearly 700 more calories than they did in 1978.

What resulted was this trend of obesity. Obesity has become an increasingly important clinical and public health challenge worldwide. According to International Obesity Taskforce estimates, there are about 1.1 billion overweight people and 350 million obese individuals worldwide. In the U.S., the prevalence of obesity has more than doubled in the past 25 years. Nearly two-thirds of adults are either overweight or obese. This number is expected two grow to alarming levels in the next decade. Childhood obesity is also on the rise.

When I went to nursing school many years ago, type 2 diabetes was known as adult onset diabetes. This was not a disease that affected children. Well, today it does. Sometime toward the end of last decade the name was changed because the disease process was changing, affecting children as well as adults. It was, therefore, re-named and today it is known as type 2 diabetes. More and more children are being diagnosed with type 2 diabetes, and from what I hear they are seeing this disease in children as young as six and seven years old. This is a serious condition with worse outcomes long-term than even type 1 diabetes.

Chapter 3
10 Things that Grandma Did

1. Grandma always cooked her own food.

Grandma cooked her food out of necessity. If she didn't cook, the family would not eat. Where I grew up in Africa, we didn't have fast foods restaurants, pizza delivery places and such things. But we had sit-down restaurants where people could eat or take-out food. When I go back to Kenya today, I find pizza places, drive-by restaurants and many fast food places as well. My grandma considered eating out a waste of money and a sign of laziness. She used to say that unless someone is traveling and away from home, there is absolutely no reason to eat out.

I happen to agree with her. When I started my weight loss journey, I found out that if I cooked my own food I could control the amount of carbohydrates, the kind of fats, as well as how much fat I put in it. The food is usually much healthier.

Today, I go to the supermarket once a week and prepare all my food for the week at home.

Research finds that people who eat out more often, particularly at fast-food restaurants, are likely to be overweight or obese. So let me ask you, how often do you eat out?

- *Three times a day?*

- *Once a day?*

- *Once a week?*

2. Grandma drank a lot of water.

Grandma was always working outside the house on her farm either tending to her crops or feeding the animals. She had cows and chickens on the farm.

She kept herself well-hydrated by drinking lots of water. I never saw her drinking fruit juices or sodas. Whenever she needed to eat something sweet, she would eat a piece of fruit, i.e., a banana, an orange, passion fruit, a mango or one of many other different fruits when in season. Now, there is nothing wrong with drinking fruit juices, but if you have to drink it, remember to drink 100% fruit juice (not from concentrate).

Also bear in mind that even 100% fruit juice is loaded with sugar; so be mindful of how much you are drinking. Remember that ½ a glass of 100% fruit juice is equivalent to one piece of fruit. I personally do not drink fruit juices. I eat the fruit itself. I also keep it to a maximum of only three different fruits per day. Fruits have sugar and if you are trying to keep your weight down, they can sabotage that effort.

Take away point: Drink at least 10 glasses of water a day.

If you ever wanted to detox your body naturally, water is the way to go. It will cleanse your body down to the cellular level and leave you feeling more alert and energized.

Helpful hint: Has anyone ever tried to sell you alkaline water claiming that alkaline water is superior to regular water? If so, save your money. If you are eating whole foods, fruits and vegetables; those foods are alkaline in nature, and you don't need to drink alkaline water to be better hydrated.

3. Grandma drank two cups of coffee or tea a day.

My grandma always started her day with a cup of tea. She also ended the work day with a cup of tea at about 5 p.m. when she was done working on the farm. She said that tea relaxed her. On cold and rainy days, she drank coffee. She seemed to think that coffee kept her warm when it was cold outside.

• *While I don't think that last statement is true, all the same, coffee and tea are good for you. I have met people who seem to think that coffee is not good for you. Coffee is a good thing. It has benefits that most people don't even know about.*

Truth be told, if you are sensitive to caffeine, I would recommend not drinking it. Some people are sensitive and it makes them hyper, jittery and some even report heart palpitations. So, if that is you, don't drink it.

Coffee and tea are naturally occurring products. Coffee is made from coffee beans and tea is made from tea leaves.

These two products are loaded with polyphenols and antioxidants that protect your immune systems and can protect you from some cancers.

• *Coffee also can lower the risk of developing erectile dysfunctions in men. Wow, who knew? Some researchers studied a group of men who had erectile dysfunctions as well as other chronic issues like heart disease, high blood pressure, overweight and obesity issues. They found that men who drunk 2-3 cups of coffee a day lowered their risk of developing erectile dysfunction.*

This is a huge plus for coffee.

Grandma also drank a lot of bone broth. This is popularly known in Kenya as "soup." If you go to a restaurant and order soup, you will be served bone broth unless you specify that you want vegetable soup or chicken soup.

This is a popular drink for women and men even to this day. It's also recommended for lactating women because it helps them produce more milk. Growing up in Kenya, I didn't know the values of bone broth. Looking at research now, it is considered a clean drink and is rich in minerals and other nutrients including calcium, magnesium, collagen, glucosamine, and chondroitin. It is also said to have anti-inflammatory properties that help protect one's immune system against viruses, bacteria and other disease causing agents.

For those trying to lose weight, bone broth is tasty, low in fat (if prepared properly), and filling without adding calories. It's also a high-octane fat burner.

4. Grandma used real cane sugar or honey in beverages.

When she drank her coffee or tea, Grandma liked it sweet but not too sweet. She always added real cane sugar to it.

- *Grandma didn't use artificial sweeteners.*

We need more research about this, but early studies are finding that these non-caloric sweeteners may disrupt the microbiome (the good bacteria community in the gut) and boost the growth of certain bacteria that triggers fat storage.

Artificial sweeteners are also highly processed and Grandma didn't do processed foods.

She never used much sugar either. She always said that too much sugar can cause diabetes. I don't think Grandma quite understood the diabetic disease process but she had a point.

- *Today we know that sugar is a carbohydrate, and, if one consumes too much of it, it turns into fat and is stored in the body; hence, most people who consume too many carbohydrates tend to be obese and obesity does cause insulin resistance, leading to type 2 diabetes.*

- *When Grandma had a cold or cough, she added honey to her tea. When she had a bad cold or one of us kids was coughing really badly, she usually gave us a teaspoonful of honey. Funny enough, it soothed our throats and calmed down the cough. A word of caution though: go easy on the added sugar.*

- *Honey has carbohydrates as well; so use it sparingly, but it has antioxidants that are good for the immune system. It's actually a better remedy for coughs than cough medicine; which most people use to soothe a hacking cough.*

- *Honey also has some healing properties, and it can kill bacteria at the back of your throat and relieve sore throats and irritation.*

- *According to the American Diabetic Society, women can have six teaspoons of added sugar per day, and men can have up to nine teaspoons per day.*

These are also known as discretionary calories. Those are calories available to a person to spend after they have already met their nutrient needs for the day. So you have to use these sparingly. However, it's there for you if you need it to loosen up the diet a little bit.

5. Grandma had a kitchen garden.

Grandma had a kitchen garden and grew her own vegetables. She always used these fresh vegetables in her foods. She had vegetables like tomatoes, cucumbers, carrots, onions, spinach, garlic, cilantro, red hot peppers and many other beneficial herbs that she used to boost the flavor in her food.

I plant tomatoes in my backyard every summer. These tomatoes have the best taste ever. There is truly a difference between just-picked vegetables and the not so fresh ones.

While it's not always possible to grow your own vegetables, one can make an effort to buy fresh vegetables from the neighborhood supermarket, the local farms in your area, the farmer's market or the flea market.

- *There's no reason to use canned or frozen fruits and vegetables when you can get fresh ones.*

- *These days one can even have fresh fruits and vegetables delivered to your home on a weekly basis.*

- *If you have to use canned vegetables, look for the ones canned in glass jars, e.g., tomatoes in a glass jar.*

6. Grandma was on the move all the time.

Grandma worked on her farm most days. She walked from one place to the other, lifted and carried things such as farm tools, cow feed, gallons of milk or water from the shed to the main house. Sometimes she moved tools up or down the hill depending on where they needed to go. She was a busy woman and never did the same thing for too long. She worked from sunrise to sundown, but she took a two or three-hour lunch break because the sun was too hot to work outside from about noon to 3 o'clock. Grandma maintained the same weight throughout her life and she never went to a gym.

I don't work on the farm like Grandma did, but I make sure I *move* a lot during my working hours. I do not go to the gym either.

I exercise for 10-20 minutes a day before heading off to work. (l lift weights and do strength training to tone up). In my house, I have a set of weights and some dumbbells as well. Sometimes I do push-ups for 5-6 minutes before taking a shower in the morning. At work, I park my car away from the building and get a 5-minute brisk walk to the office. While at work, I take the stairs instead of riding the elevator. I walk during my lunch break and by the end of the day, I have had a workout just like Grandma did.

You too can do like Grandma did. Aim to exercise at least 20 minutes every day. Use the weights around your house. Lifting gallons of milk or water can do the trick. Better yet, invest in some dumbbells or some weights and multi-task. Lift some weights as you watch your favorite TV show.

Get rid of your recliner, and in its place have a stair master. You will be glad you did. A daily exercise routine is worth its weight in gold.

Don't ever say, you don't have time to exercise.

Being physically active does not mean that you have to spend two hours in the gym every day.

When people hear the word "exercise," they immediately think of a physical activity that is planned, structured and repetitive. Many people hate that and they will come up with all kinds of excuses why they cannot exercise. They might say they have no time to do it, lack the money for a gym membership; some say they hate to sweat or to go out to the gym. I can assure you that Grandma didn't go to the gym. Actually, the way she did it—by moving most of her waking hours—is the best way to stay physically active.

Studies show that people who sit all day in their jobs have a 40% greater chance of dying sooner than those who move about during their working hours.

Even if you exercise once a day in the gym before heading to work, what you do for the rest of the day matters a lot too. So, don't just sit there; get some short bouts of standing and physical activity to break-up the prolonged sitting. You need to find reasons to get up from your desk and move. Walking, even for five minutes at a time, makes a huge difference.

Benefits of daily exercise:

- *You lose weight, even as you sleep, long after the exercise session is over, especially if you incorporate strength training with cardio.*

- *Exercise decreases your waist circumference, (abdominal obesity), and this is the type of obesity that places people at risk for heart disease and type 2 diabetes more than any other type of obesity.*

  If you stand up straight and cannot see your toes while standing up, you have abdominal obesity and need to pay close attention. This is bad for you. You've got belly fat.

- *You can improve that muffin top and the middle-age sag with strength training (also known as resistance training).*

- *Exercise also spurs the formation of new brain cells and prevents diseases like dementia and Alzheimer—something even scientist had long thought was impossible. Exercise improves cognitive functions.*

- *It prevents certain types of cancer like breast and colon cancer.*

- *It decreases symptoms of depression and anxiety and improves mood.*

- *It prevents early death from heart disease, high blood pressure and strokes.*

- *It reduces bad cholesterol and prevents type 2 diabetes.*

- *You may have heard of people falling and dying while trying to get in and out of the shower or just trying to sit on a commode. Exercise prevents falls and improves balance, especially in older adults by improving functional health: the ability to wash, and get in and out of the shower without mishaps.*

- *Exercise can help with weight loss particularly when combined with reduced calories.*

- *Exercise helps you sleep better.*

The list goes on and on.

Grandma was physically fit up to a few days before her death. She died of pneumonia. She thought she had a bad cold and instead of going to the hospital, she went to bed. She passed away in her sleep.

What is physical fitness anyway?

Is it looking skinny?

Is it the number on the scale that determines how fit one is?

Physical fitness is the ability to carry out daily tasks with vigor and alertness without undue fatigue and with ample energy to enjoy them. Grandma did that until the day she passed away.

> Take your time and do it the right way.
> Grandma always said,
> "There is no short-cut to any place worth going."

The best way to lose weight is to reduce at a rate of one-half to two pounds per week.

7. Grandma baked and bought sweets on special occasions only.

Whether grandma did this because she was trying to save money or for some other reason, she never bought sweets or baked cakes unless it was a major holiday or special occasion. Growing up, the only chance I got to eat cake was at weddings.

Now if we had company or if a special holiday was coming up, Grandma would buy sodas, juices and scones and other baked goods for the occasion. She never bought those things to have around the house.

I have a friend who was on a diet to lose weight, but every time she went to the store and found candy, chocolate bars and other sweets on sale she would buy them and keep them in her house. Every now and then she would take a bag of candy to the office. When she had a bad day at work, she would come home and consume large amounts of those sweets.

I would say, do like Grandma did. Don't buy or keep sugary snacks in the house. It's difficult to resist eating it if it's right there. If you go to a party and they are serving cake and other sweets, eat some but do not take any home. Stop buying candy, donuts and bagels for people at work. They don't need them either.

8. Grandma ate a lot of whole foods legumes and pulses.

Although Grandma occasionally ate meats, she mostly ate legumes, pulses (dry legumes), root vegetables, grains, nuts, eggs, fruits, vegetables and dairy products. She was not a vegetarian by any means but meat was not a large part of her diet.

Most of her meals contained legumes and pulses of all colors, flavors and textures. She consumed porridge made with ground grains like sorghum, oats, wheat, corn and millet. For carbohydrates, she consumed mostly whole foods like plantains, yams, sweet potatoes, white potatoes, corn, cassava, pumpkin and arrowroot.

She added a lot of vegetables to her meals: carrots, cabbage, spinach, kale, collard greens, tomatoes and others. She ate nuts and fruits such as avocado and peanuts for healthy fats. We had avocado trees, peanuts and macadamia nuts growing on our farm.

We too can eat like Grandma did. This will ensure that we are eating clean every single day. These foods are easily accessible in local food markets. You don't have to have a farm to eat clean.

It's true that whole foods take longer to cook, but you will be eating less harmful products by avoiding processed foods. Take time to prepare meals; you are worth it.

Invest in a slow cooker, and make it your best friend. This way, you can cook those foods that take a while to cook like dry legumes and other grains. Put some of these dry beans in the pot, and they can cook while you are at work or while you are sleeping.

There are so many ways you can include whole foods in your diet. Cook a whole bunch of food, refrigerate and eat it for two to three days so you don't have to cook every day. You can also freeze the food in small packages and eat it for two to three weeks.

- Use whole foods like legumes, i.e., beans, chickpeas and lentils. Grains like quinoa, spelt, teff, amaranth, farro, barley and bulgur have a lot of fiber so they keep you full for a longer period of time.

  They have both complex carbohydrates and proteins not to mention a lot of beneficial vitamins and minerals

- These complex carbohydrates have a low glycemic index which means that they breakdown slowly and hence slow down digestion and absorption.

- Slow digestion and absorption keeps your metabolism working hard and keeps your body supplied with energy for a longer period of time.

- Legumes decrease your bad cholesterol (LDL) because they are generally low in fat.

- Legumes will definitely help you lose weight and keep it off.

I encourage you to do like Grandma did and eat more legumes instead of meat, especially red meat.

9. Grandma breastfed all her children.

Grandma breastfed all her children. She always said that good health starts at birth. We can go even further and say good health starts before conception with the woman taking care of her health and fitness three to six months before she conceives.

A woman should be at a healthy weight before conceiving. She should take a multivitamin and folic acid to prepare the body for conception and the birth of a healthy baby.

Once conception takes place, a woman should continue eating healthy and continue exercising. She should not try new exercises while pregnant but should continue with what her body is used to doing. We don't want anyone getting injured trying new things at this time. Once the baby is born, unless contraindicated, babies do well when fed the mother's milk, the way God intended it.

- *Breastfed babies maintain a strong immune system.*

- *They do not get as many colds, ear infections, and allergies to foods as non-breastfed infants.*

- *They also maintain a healthy body weight as they*

grow older (unlike formula-fed babies).

- They have fewer endocrine problems such as advanced bone age and early onset of puberty which seems to lead to overweight children.

- *Breast milk is free; so it will help you save money as well.*

Grandma also prepared all her babies' foods. She never fed her babies any commercially prepared foods. My mom did the same. I followed in my grandma's and my mom's footsteps. Even though my kids were born in America, I could never bring myself to feed them store bought baby food. I would have cringed at the thought of feeding them food bought in a jar knowing very well that it was not fresh, and probably had additives, coloring and preservatives. Commercially prepared baby food was unheard of growing up in Kenya. Every woman I knew prepared her own baby food. It was usually baked or boiled without any salt or oil added. Once cooked, she would puree the food and feed it to her babies.

I did the same thing baking and boiling food for all my babies. Once fully cooked, I would put the food in a blender and puree it. I fed my kids legumes, pumpkin, sweet potatoes, carrots, peas, mashed bananas, papayas, watermelon, and avocado. I would taste the food before feeding it to my kids, and it was fresh, clean and tasted **very** good.

When the babies turned one year or so, my grandma

would stop breast feeding and give them whole milk. I grew up on whole milk as well and only started drinking skim milk in my early twenties.

One personal observation I have made since coming to this country is that there are a lot of children with ADHD (Attention Deficit Hyperactivity Disorder). My whole life growing up in Kenya, I never met one kid with ADHD. Even to this day when I go back to visit, I still don't see children with this disorder. ADHD was unknown to me until I came to this country. Although not research based, I personally think this disorder might be tied to the environment and the food we feed our children. If you look closely at what healthcare providers recommend as a ADHD diet, it's nothing new. They recommend eating clean, avoiding foods with additives like MSG, nitrites, yellow or red food coloring, and skipping foods high in simple sugars or simple carbohydrates. I suggest you do like Grandma did and prepare your own baby food using fresh and whole foods without any additives. Make a lot and refrigerate the food for up to three days so you don't have to cook every day.

I also noticed lately that people are giving their children low fat milk instead of whole milk. The fat in the milk and some cholesterol are building blocks for growing bodies.

Kids really need whole milk because their brains and bodies are still developing and growing. Once they reach the ages of 20-25, they can switch to low fat and skim milk.

10. Grandma slept a total of eight hours a night.

Grandma always said that a day is made up of 12 hours. She always said that God made darkness for a reason, and when it gets dark humans are supposed to sleep. On our farm, even the cows and the chickens were asleep by 9 p.m. Grandma went to bed at the same time every day and, can I tell you something? She woke up at the same time every morning. Grandma never used an alarm clock and she always woke up at 5 a.m. on the dot every morning.

When your body is fully rested, you don't need an alarm clock.

If you train your body to go to sleep at the same time every day, you will wake up alert and energized. This is true even for those who work odd shifts like evening and night shifts.

With adequate sleep your body is also less stressed and you produce less of the stress hormone "cortisol," and this makes you more likely to maintain a healthy body weight.

- When people are stressed, they eat more and they also do not care what they eat. They consume a lot of the bad foods like simple sugars and bad fats. Their bodies also produce massive amounts of the stress hormone that causes the liver to produce even more sugar especially when they sleep. This is usually a risk factor for developing type 2 diabetes.

- In short, get enough sleep and, please avoid sleeping in. Believe it or not, sleeping in is bad for your health. It can cause weight gain, even for a healthy person who exercises regularly. It can cause heart disease, slow down your cognitive functions, decrease your vocabulary and worsen depressive symptoms. Not good.

- Sleeping in stresses the body and leaves you feeling even more tired and not well-rested.

- By the way, sleeping in even on weekends can stress your body too. So, just get up as usual and take a nap later in the day if feeling tired.

- Train your body to sleep at the same time, and wake up at the same time most days even on the weekend.

- Always aim to get 7-8 hours of sleep a day for adults 18 years and older. Sleeping more than nine hours may be bad for your health. The exceptions are teenagers and children who can sleep more.

- **If you suffer from shift work disorder, instead of taking medication to help you sleep when off duty or to stay awake while working at night, you might try changing your job. Work during the day and sleep at night. You will be glad you did it and your body will thank you too.**

Chapter 4
10 Plus One Things that Grandma Didn't Do

1. Grandma didn't juice her fruits or vegetables.

Grandma would never, ever juice her fruits or vegetables, and she never bought fruit juices. Whenever she wanted fruit, she ate the fruit itself. She ate different kinds of fruits when in season: Oranges, bananas, passion fruit, pineapples, apples, plums, and peaches were among those she enjoyed.

When you eat whole fruits without juicing them, you get a lot of vitamins and fiber.

Fiber is very beneficial in many ways:

- It keeps you full for a longer time period; hence, you consume less food.

- Fiber keeps bad cholesterol down and well regulated.

- Fiber helps with bowel elimination and keeps you regular. It's a wonderful natural treatment for constipation.

- Fiber prevents colon cancers.

A word of caution: Fruit juices have way too much sugar. They are calorie dense.

2. Grandma didn't do smoothies.

While there is nothing wrong with smoothies, my grandma didn't drink them. No smoothies for me either, because I like to eat my food, not drink it.

I recommend that people chew their food unless they have no teeth or have another reason like being on a puree or a liquid diet.

Smoothies are wonderful if you are a <u>*triathlete*</u> *and in good physical shape. I don't recommend smoothies for people trying to lose weight, because they contain way too many carbs and are high in calories.*

People who make smoothies tend to put 3-4 fruits in the smoothie to make it taste good. Fruits are loaded with carbohydrates and they might hinder your weight loss efforts.

The Benefits of Chewing Your Food

- You tend to eat slower, allowing your stomach to communicate with your brain sending it feelings of satiety. As a result, you consume less food.

- Once the food gets to the stomach, more breaking down of the food is needed, so digestion and absorption are slower. This keeps you full longer so you consume less food.

- The process of chewing food is an exercise in itself, and it keeps your facial joints well lubricated.

- Chewing promotes blood supply to the brain and keeps you alert, improves cognition, actually decreases the risks of dementia and slows down the progression of Alzheimer's disease.

3. Grandma didn't drink instant coffee.

On Grandma's farm she grew tea and coffee among other things. When she had time she would pick the coffee beans and take them to the coffee factory for processing. She also picked the tea leaves which she took to the tea factory.

Sometimes she dried her own coffee beans herself, roasted them and made her own coffee grounds. You can do that with coffee, but with tea it's a bit more complicated. She left the tea to the experts, and she went to the tea factory once a month to buy her tea bags. When I travel to Kenya, I make a trip to the tea factory and buy enough tea leaves to last me a year or so. I can assure you this tea tastes different, and it is better than store-bought teas.

You can prepare your own coffee as well. There are stores that sell coffee beans and can grind them for you if desired.

If you have ever tasted freshly ground coffee, you know it's very flavorful; it tastes good and the aroma is pleasing.

Instant coffee is different. It has a bitter taste and is less caffeinated. It does not smell nor taste like coffee.

Grandma hated the taste of instant coffee, and she knew it was processed because it tasted and smelled different from the real deal.

> *Instant coffee contains the harmful chemical Cafesol found in all coffees. Cafesol is a substance that increases bad cholesterol.*

When you brew ground coffee, cafesol is filtered out with a strainer, but with instant coffee there is no way to filter it out. *There's also a high amount of acrylamide which occurs naturally when certain foods are heated to very high temperatures. Acrylamide has been shown to cause cancer in animals. It can also cause nerve damage in humans according to the Food and Drug Administration. Instant coffee has much higher amounts of this substance than ground coffee.*

Brew your coffee and do not drink instant coffee. When it comes to substances that are not good for you, instant coffee is as bad as processed foods.

4. Grandma didn't use liquid or powdered coffee creamers.

Grandma used whole milk in her tea and coffee. I know most people do not use milk in their coffee and prefer to use creamers. Some of these creamers really taste good in coffee. However, they are highly processed and not really good for you.

They are mostly non-dairy and have more than 10 ingredients. This number shows that they are highly processed.

Most liquid creamers are made with water, high fructose corn syrup, cotton seed oils, sodium caseinate (a milk derivative) and other ingredients.

Powdered creamers are even worse because—on top of what I have already mentioned—they add artificial colors, artificial flavors and trans fat. Trans fat is the worst kind of fat any human can eat. In my opinion if you eat trans fat, you might as well eat poison. It's not good for healthy clean eating and definitely not good for weight management.

- Do like Grandma did; use whole milk and work your way to skim milk for your coffee. Try switching gradually from whole milk to 1% milk. You will get used to the difference in flavor, and in no time, you too can start enjoying a healthier cup of coffee. I promise you with time you will like it as much as you like your current choice of coffee creamer.

- Milk is minimally processed; it provides some vitamins, it's low in sodium and lower in calories.

If you don't like to use milk like Grandma did, you can use something that is closer to milk and blends in well with coffee. It's also much creamier.

- o Half-and-half is far less processed, and it contains real dairy products.

- o Another product you can use is heavy cream.

  The two products above contain whole foods and have little to no carbohydrates. They are made from pasteurized Grade A milk and cream.

- By the way, dairy fat is actually not bad for you. If you eat 1-2 servings of dairy products a day, you will be fine.

- The milk you use in coffee is a really small amount and should not even count. You can count it as a free item.

- It is the trans fat, the processed stuff, the corn syrup and added sugar that make creamers the bad guys. Those are the ones you need to worry about.

- So, if you want your coffee creamier and you really don't want to use milk, you can safely use the heavy creams or half-and-half.

5. Grandma didn't smoke, drink alcohol or use illicit drugs.

Grandma never smoked.

She didn't drink alcohol.

She didn't use any kind of illicit drugs or addictive prescription drugs. **Grandma was a smart woman.**

Grandma always said that if you treat your body right by feeding it well and not using addictive substances, your body will treat you well in return.

Can I confide in you about something? Growing up I didn't know that women smoked. I never saw a woman smoke until I was a teenager and went to the city to visit my older sister. I thought that smoking was a guy's thing.

You may know that less than 3% of Americans are:

- *active enough*
- *healthy eaters*
- *non-smokers and*
- *at a healthy weight and healthy percentage of body fat*

Less than 3%! This is according to a study published in Mayo Clinic Proceedings in April 2016.

This is shocking.

The study was conducted from August 2013 through January 2016.

It is remarkable that less than 3% of the population meets the goal. The factors mentioned above are the four most important elements of a heart-healthy lifestyle. Combined, these are what is promoted by the American Heart Association (AHA). They have made this a strategic focus as an impact goal for the year 2020 and beyond.

We definitely have a long way to go.

I am surprised when I see doctors and nurses smoking. They have first-hand information about what happens when you treat your body this way. They take care of patients on their death beds who wish they never smoked. They see it every single day and still light up when they go out to take breaks.

I even worry more when I see overweight and obese individuals smoking. That is two strikes against your health.

Remember, heart disease is the leading cause of death in United States.

More women are dying from this disease than men. In fact, it's the number one killer of women, and the symptoms are more difficult to identify.

The National Institute of Health estimates that by the year 2030—less than 15 years from when this was published—40% of the population will have some form of heart disease.

The rates are expected to be higher for African American women.

6. Grandma didn't do gluten-free diets.

The gluten-free diet is another area where people are confused. Some people eat gluten-free foods in an effort to lose weight. Others eat it because they have heard of the horrors of eating gluten.

Gluten is the alcohol-soluble part of the wheat protein. It is present in foods such as wheat, barley, rye and (to a minor degree) oats. Gluten is found in many of our food products: cereal, bread, pasta and to some extent on some of the enteric-coated medicines.

I eat gluten just like my mom and my grandma did. It's never made me sick, and I don't need to start a gluten-free diet now in my 50s.

It is hard to stay on a gluten-free diet, and, if you don't have to, why do it? Gluten-free does not mean better weight control, and it doesn't necessarily mean healthier foods.

There are people who should avoid gluten: people with a diagnoses of **Celiac disease** and those who are **gluten-sensitive** or **gluten-intolerant**. Gluten does not affect everybody, but, for those whom it does, it can cause some bad outcomes.

I think the confusion occurs when we start talking about gluten-sensitivity. This affects a lot of people in different ways and sometimes the symptoms are very vague. Some people experience gastro-intestinal disturbances such as bloating, diarrhea and acid reflux. These symptoms can also result from other causes or diseases and may not be due to consuming gluten.

If you are unsure whether or not to eliminate gluten from your diet, check with your primary care provider. There is a test for gluten-sensitivity. You can take the test and clarify whether or not you are gluten-sensitive.

Don't put yourself on a gluten-free diet just because others are doing it. You will be cheating yourself of some very valuable nutrients found in bulgur, wheat, oats, oat bran, barley and rye.

Soluble fibers found in these foods are used by the body to reduce bad cholesterol. The fiber found in gluten-containing products also blocks the absorption of cholesterol and other fats (triglycerides) by creating a gel-like substance that slows down the movement of the food in the gut. This gel-like substance coats the intestines and slows absorption of fats and sugars. That is good for diabetic patients. This fiber is also helpful in weight management by increasing satiation and satiety. You will miss all these benefits and many more if you put yourself on a dietary restriction that you didn't need in the first place.

If you still insist on a gluten-free diet, talk with your health care provider and see if and how you need to supplement your diet. You may need a multivitamin and a multi-mineral as well psyllium (a soluble fiber) to give you the same benefit as the gluten-containing foods.

7. Grandma didn't do microwaves.

Almost every household today has a microwave and it's hard to imagine life without one. My grandma grew up without a microwave in the house, and she was used to baking, boiling or grilling her food. Quite frankly, she was deathly afraid of microwaves. She would never eat anything made or warmed in a microwave. In those days, signs were posted to warn pregnant women not to enter a room because a microwave might be in use.

My grandma thought that microwaved food was warmed up by some kind of radiation energy which she thought would spill into the food. As far as she was concerned, microwaved food was poison.

You might think that her fear was unfounded, but, with the current focus on clean eating, there are some people who are turning away from using microwaves to cook or warm food. I am not one of those people, but lately I too have cut down on using the microwave as much as I once did.

> One reason for rethinking microwave use is the on-going theory claiming that microwaved food does not contain the same chemical structure of nutrients as that which is cooked the conventional way. The claims state that the microwave energy uses the water in the vegetables/food by bouncing the water bubbles back and forth to warm or cook it, destroying the nutrient

structure of the food and leaving it less nutritious.

One thing is for sure: People don't pay attention to the containers that they use to warm the food. Many people use plastic containers which contain a chemical known as BPA (Bisphenol A) that leaks into the food and is known to cause serious health problems like cancer and many other endocrine health issues.

If we were to test everybody's urine today, mine included, 95% of us would have detectable, significant levels of BPA in our system. BPA is one of the known endocrine-disrupting chemicals in our environment.

Use paper plates or china plates in the microwave, not plastic. And on the same note, hand wash your plastics and don't put them in the dish washer even if they tell you it's safe to put plastics on the top rack.

With so many toxins in our environment today, our job is to lessen exposure to them as much as possible. That is why we need to cook our food like Grandma did. Boil it, bake it or grill it.

Avoid microwave popcorn. Air pop your popcorn. The lining of the paper container used in microwave popcorn is known to have BPA as well, and the fake butter turns into bad fat that is not healthy for human consumption. Also you will want to avoid the high salt content in microwave popcorn as well.

8. Grandma didn't eat anything she could not read or pronounce.

Grandma was not very learned, but she could read and write. When growing up where I came from, they didn't see a need to send their girls to school. Most girls got married at a young age and became homemakers. My grandma could only read at the fourth grade level.

However, Grandma took pride in her ability to read and write. She liked to read everything she got her hands on: labels, newspapers and other written materials. Grandma did not eat anything she could not read or pronounce.

When reading product ingredients, she avoided anything too complicated or the ones that she didn't recognize as real foods.

We should have the same mentality that Grandma had.

Get in the habit of reading food labels. If a label has ingredients you cannot pronounce, please stay away from that food. Words that are too difficult to understand or ones that don't sound like real foods indicate that these products are most likely processed.

If a product has more than five ingredients, most likely it is processed and you need to leave it alone.

9. Grandma didn't do diets.

Grandma didn't do any diets and she maintained a health body weight all her adult years. If you are on a diet, don't feel badly; keep reading and figure out how your diet compares to Grandma's healthy living. I also want you to think about your diet long-term. Do you think this is something you will do for the rest of your life? If your answer is "yes," then continue doing what you are doing, but if your answer is "NO" pay close attention.

Studies show that people who diet fail 95% of the time. Most diets are not realistic, and people don't like to be controlled and restricted. Diets are not fun, and they go against human nature. People get tired of tracking every morsel they eat. Nobody wants to live on a 1000 calories a day for the rest of his or her life. People like to be in control, and they love to be free—free from dieting.

Most people who diet either give up after a few days, or they lose the weight and resume their old habits only to gain all the weight back.

You know why Grandma didn't do any diets? She didn't need to. Eating right is not complicated. The truth about diets is that they don't work long-term. How many people do you know who wake up every morning excited about counting calories and tracking everything they eat?

Grandma didn't do detox diets either. She didn't

do any protein shakes or protein bars. Knowing my grandma, there was no way she would have consumed any of that.

Do you know why protein shakes and protein bars do not taste good? They are highly processed and not very palatable. Nobody wants to eat that kind of food for too long.

We all now know that diets don't work. With that said, I don't want you to diet. I would prefer you make good choices that you can live with for the rest of your life.

- Good health is more than a number on the scale.

- Good health is not about looking skinny.

It's about how well your body functions. That means functioning without excessive fatigue in performing the activities of daily living: playing with your kids, cleaning your house, moving furniture, going up and down the stairs, performing your job, doing yard work, walking your dog and other daily activities that are required of you.

It's about decreasing risk factors for cancer, heart and vascular diseases, osteoarthritis and type 2 diabetes.

If you adopt a lifestyle where you drink 10 glasses of water a day, eat whole foods, avoid processed foods and load your plate with fruits and vegetables of different colors, you will naturally train your body to crave healthy foods and you won't need to be on a diet. This will be a lifestyle you can live with and maintain.

I must tell you, though, I lost my way for a while in my early 30s after my younger daughter was born. I gained a lot of weight. I was 50 pounds over my ideal body weight and kept that for 15 years.

Then I went back to my old eating habits:

➢ Eating whole foods, a few fruits and lots of vegetables

➢ drinking adequate amounts of water

➢ cooking my own food

➢ moving more

I lost forty-nine pounds. That was three years ago and I have kept the weight off to date. This is a lifestyle I will keep for the rest of my life.

Anybody can do this. It's not complicated and not time consuming. I am free to live my life and enjoy the journey of weight management.

Freedom is: free to eat and live your life and to live your life and eat.

10. The plus one thing that Grandma didn't do, But I want you to do.

I mentioned in the beginning that Grandma worked on the farm. That means she was outdoors most of the day. She also lived in a warm and sunny country, Kenya, Africa.

Grandma did not take vitamin D. However, I want you to take it. It's sold over the counter and it's cheap.

> *But before you start taking vitamin D, talk with your health care provider and get a blood test to check your levels. Although this is not part of your routine annual physical work-up, it's cheap to do and can be added to your routine blood test. Simply tell your doctor that you are concerned and that you would like to know what your vitamin D level is.*

Vitamin D is actually not a vitamin. It's more like a hormone. Your body can make it in the right environment. Exposure to the sun is one of the most important conditions for your body to make this wonderful vitamin. Grandma didn't take it because her body made enough as a result of her lifestyle and location.

Vitamin D is used in your body to maintain proper calcium levels so your heart, other body muscles and bones can work and develop properly.

There are people who are at risk for vitamin D deficiency and need to talk with their doctors to have this checked. With low levels chances of developing osteoporosis at a young age are very common along with a whole host of other possible bad outcomes. These include conditions like Alzheimer's disease and other dementias.

Take home nuggets:

Vitamin D is not harmful when taken in low doses of about 700-1000 international units per day.

Vitamin D deficiency is associated with a poor health status.

Get tested.

At risk individuals:

> *Dark skinned people in general are at risk for vitamin D deficiency. Your skin color blocks the sunlight from getting into your body.*

> *Dark skinned people who have moved from warm weather countries to the western world do not get adequate sunshine in the winter months.*

> *Women who are veiled. Their skin is not exposed to sunshine.*

> *People who work indoors with UV protected windows.*

> *People who wear sunscreen.*

People who take antacids for indigestion or acid re-flux. These substances prevent absorption of vitamin D and calcium as well.

People who don't drink milk.

Home bound individuals or those living in nursing homes.

People who have had multiple bone fractures.

Infants, pregnant women and lactating women.

Women who suffer from pre-menstrual mood syndrome.

People who take seizure medications.

People who are obese. This vitamin is stored in the body fat (it's a fat soluble vitamin), and obese people need more of it.

The benefits of vitamin D are numerous. Research is still on-going about this vitamin. Some of the beneficial elements mentioned are:

- Patients who suffer with pre-menstrual mood syndrome do better when taking vitamin D.

- People with Alzheimer's and other dementias also do better when taking this vitamin.

- People who suffer from depression improve their mood when taking this vitamin.

- People who take vitamin D report fewer symptoms of osteoporosis than those who don't take it. They also report fewer bone fractures and lower risks of falling because of better balance and agility.

- The bones and muscles work better when taking vitamin D.

- Vitamin D is said to decrease risk of developing some cancers like colorectal and breast cancer.

- Vitamin D improves symptoms of myalgia (muscle pain) and fibromyalgia (a chronic pain syndrome).

More research findings about this wonderful vitamin are coming out in the year 2017. Stay tuned.

Chapter 5
Clean & Healthy Eating

Clean and healthy eating is not complicated. You too can do like Grandma did.

You don't have to pay money to have someone tell you what you need to eat. Simply do like Grandma did and you will have no trouble keeping your weight under control and living a healthy, long life.

Remember, nothing is sweeter than good health.

Clean healthy eating will add years to your life and life to your years.

Always remember:

> He who takes medication and neglects diet wastes the skill of his doctor.
>
> A Chinese proverb

Chapter 6
Your Drink of Choice

Your drink of choice should always be H_2O.

If you are having trouble committing to a healthy diet, start slowly, and just change one thing. Begin by drinking 16 ounces of water before breakfast, lunch and dinner. Your drink of choice should be water. Try it: It will change your life.

Alice W. Munyua

Chapter 7
How to Make Healthy Habits Stick

1. **Block anxiety**. While organizing your life and overhauling your diet to achieve healthy goals is good for you, it can cause a lot of anxiety. The best way to handle that stress is to plan ahead. Be prepared. Pick a night once a week or on your day off to plan your meals for the week. Make a shopping list as well and post it on the refrigerator so the whole family knows what's for dinner every night of the week.

2. **Think small**. Tackling one small goal before moving to the next one is a great way to break old habits and develop new ones. So, instead of going on a strict diet, consider simple replacements, i.e., substituting one can of soda with a glass of water. Replace one snack with a piece of fruit or go for a walk daily for 10 to 15 minutes. If you work on small goals for several days to a week, you are more than likely to achieve them than if you change everything all at once.

- For example, think about this: You go on a liquid diet for 21 days to lose 21 pounds. You didn't gain all this weight in one month and you didn't develop all those bad habits in one week. It happened slowly. You can change bad habits just as easily as you develop them. Think small and go slowly.

3. **Get motivated.** Collect inspirational quotes from books and magazine articles. Get pictures of yourself when you felt and looked your best. If you don't have a picture of you when you looked your best, then cut an image from a magazine of someone who looks like the ideal you, and place a picture of your face on it. Put the picture and your quotes on the refrigerator door, your computer screen, IPad screen or the mirror on your bathroom wall. Put them somewhere you will be able to see the inspirational quotes and look at the picture on a daily basis. This will remind you every day what you are working toward.

4. **Set an end goal in mind.** Beat your burn-out by keeping your eyes on the goal or prize. Write out what it means for you to be your ideal best. For instance, one might say, "I want to be someone who is lean, strong and physically active," or "I want to be healthy enough to participate in the 5k walk for diabetes," or "I want to be healthy enough to watch my granddaughter graduate from college or get married." Once you write your goals down, place them on a bedside table and read them out loud at night before going to bed and every

morning when you awaken. This will prevent you from getting burn out and quitting on yourself.

5. **Watch your words.** Become aware of that come out of your mouth. This is where many people fail. The battle lies more in what comes out of your mouth than what goes into it. Start listening to the words you say about yourself. Ask yourself, "Is this the type of thing I would ever say to somebody else?" If you cannot say it to someone else, why would you say it to yourself or about yourself even if you were just joking? Remember, the power of life and death is in the tongue.

You might catch yourself say words like:

o I cannot eat that; I will gain weight if I do.

o I have a slow metabolism; it runs in my family.

o I gain 10 pounds just by looking at cake.

o I can't just eat one cookie; I have to have twelve.

o I guess I will always be fat. Why bother exercising?

o Deep down inside of me, there is a skinny person, but I hold her off with ice cream.

      o Losing weight is so hard; I cannot do it.

      o I was a big baby anyway; I will always be big.

Consider turning some of these negatives into self-empowering positives.

Here are some examples:

      o I choose to eat things that are healthy.

      o I choose healthy activities.

      o I choose to put only healthy things into my body.

Say something positive or don't say anything at all.

Always ask yourself, do your words nurture you, or do they put you down by taking control away from you? Do your words empower you, or do they inhibit your success?

If you want a positive outcome, you have to use words to set positive expectations. This is called *the power of positive thinking* or *the power of positive suggestive thoughts*.

Chapter 8
Take Home Points

Here is some evidence of toxins in our environment:

- *Nobody is able to explain the increased rates of type 1 diabetes and thyroid disorders in the community.*

- *There have been disturbing increases in testicular, prostate, breast, ovarian and endometrial cancer— more than ever before.*

- *The number of miscarriages has risen.*

- *Increased rates of infertility are being reported.*

- *Many more health issues are emerging in our societies today.*

To lessen exposure to environmental toxins, we need to err on the side of caution and reduce the use of plastic containers and canned foods as much as possible. Buy foods that are packed in glass jars instead of the cans.

Drink from a glass *whenever possible and keep water in glass jugs.* If you have to drink from a plastic bottle, don't leave it in a warm or hot area like the inside of a car.

Make the slow cooker your best friend and cook those foods that take a long time to cook. Use your slow cooker to prepare foods like dry beans instead of buying the canned ones.

Get tested and take vitamin D if you have a deficiency!

Last but not least, simply eat like Grandma did.

Chapter 9

Do You Need One-on-One Help?

The author, Alice W. Munyua, is a Board Certified Family Nurse Practitioner, a health coach and a diabetic educator.

If you need personal dietary help or have any medical concerns and want to know what you need to do about them, the author can help. You can text your concerns to (919) 593-3812 or call and leave a voice message, and she will get back to you within 24 hours.

For more detailed one-on-one help, please hire Alice as a consultant or donate something to one of the missions she supports. You can use your Health Care Flexible Spending plan.

You can rest assured that the author will never advise you to do anything contrary to what your doctor tells you to do. You may get a different take on things, but you will be referred back to check with your health care provider. The information in this book is only supplemental to what you are doing with your doctors to fill in the gaps where nutrition is needed.

Remember the Chinese proverb:

Don't just take the medicine and neglect the diet.

Chapter 10

About the Author

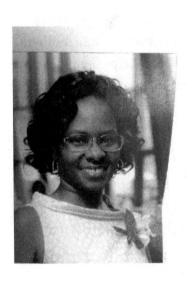

Alice W. Munyua is a graduate of Duke University School of Nursing and is a Board Certified Family Nurse Practitioner. She is actively employed in state government in North Carolina and teaches diabetic management and does weight management consultations as well.

The author has used these very ideas discussed in this book to lose a total of 49 pounds a little over three years ago and has managed to keep the weight off to date. She has helped hundreds of other people with weight control.

Highest accomplishment: Alice W. Munyua is the recipient of the 2015 Duke University School of Nursing Humanitarian Award for lifelong commitment to improving health care in her community as well as oversees in Nairobi, Kenya. She works with single mothers and women afflicted with HIV. She helps them develop business ideas to sustain themselves and their families financially.

By investing in this book, you will reward yourself with a lifelong gift of good health and well-being. You will also change someone else's life for the better. The money made from sales of this book is used to fund medical mission trips for the author to assist impoverished women and children in Kenya.

This is the gift that keeps on giving.